All About
MANAGING INCONTINENCE

By Laura Flynn R.N., B.N., M.B.A., in consultation with her nurse educator associates and physicians who assisted in contributing and editing.

Our thanks also guidelines provided by the Joint Commission on Accreditation of Home Care Organizations, the Wound Ostomy Continence Nurses (WOCN) Association, members of the Canadian Association of Enterostomal Nurses and the National Association for Continence.

ISBN No: 978 1 896616 78 0

The publisher, Mediscript Communications Inc., acknowledges the financial support of the Government of Canada through the Canadian Book Fund for our publishing activities.

Printed in Canada

www.mediscript.net

Book and Front Cover design by:
Brian Adamson, www.AdamsonGraphics.net

MI1002010

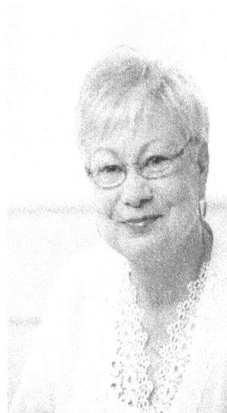

CONTENTS

INTRODUCTION

This book provides basic, non controversial and trusted information that can help a wide spectrum of readers.

The primary objective of the information is to help a person provide effective quality care to a loved one or someone in his or her care.

After reading this material you will have greater confidence in your caregiving role and will know what to do to help the incontinent person. Equally important, you will better understand the many aspects of incontinence in older people.

All the information is reliable and was written by a group of eminent nurse educators who ensured all the information complies with best practice guidelines and satisfies the various accreditation and regulatory bodies. Because there is so much unreliable information on the internet, you can be assured the "All About" publications are HON (Health On the Net) certified.

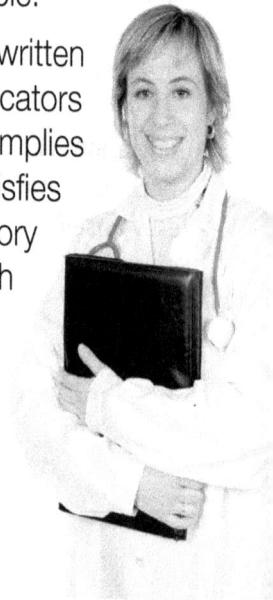

This book can be an invaluable aid to:

- A caregiver caring for a relative or friend
- A health worker seeking a reference aid
- A patient or person suffering from incontience
- Any person involved in health care wishing to expand his or her knowledge

---

SOMETHING TO THINK ABOUT...

Man's greatest need is to love and,
in turn, to love others.

Anonymous

AN IMPORTANT MESSAGE
FROM THE PUBLISHER

Each person's treatment, advice, medical aids, physical therapy and other approaches to health care are unique and highly dependant upon the diagnosis and overall assessment by the medical team.

We emphasize therefore that the information within this book is not a substitute for the advice and treatment from a health care professional.

This book provides generic information concerning the issues around incontinence and common sense, well-established care practices for people with this condition.

With all this in mind, the publishers and authors disclaim any responsibility for any adverse effects resulting directly or indirectly from the suggestions contained within this book or from any misunderstanding of the content on the part of the reader.

HAVE YOU HEARD

The following are actual bumper stickers:

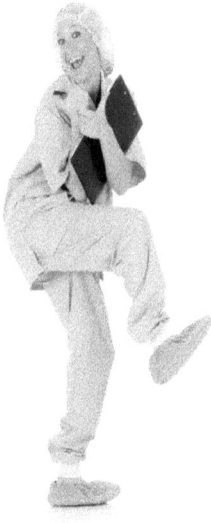

- If you don't like the news, go out and make some.

- Ever stop to think and forget to start again?

- Real women don't have hot flashes; they have power surges.

- Caution: I drive like you do.

Source: www.funnymail.com

HOW MUCH DO YOU KNOW?

It helps to figure out how much you know before you start. In this way you will have an idea as to the gaps in your knowledge prior to reading the content. Please circle to indicate the best answer. Remember, at this stage, you are not expected to know all the answers:

1. Incontinence is a disease.

a) True

b) False

2. Incontinence affects very few people.

a) True

b) False

3. Incontinence affects people of all ages.

a) True

b) False

4. Once you become incontinent, nothing can be done about it.

a) True

b) False

5. Incontinence is only a "woman's" problem.

a) True

b) False

6. Electrical stimulation is used to treat:

a) Nocturia

b) Stress and urge incontinence

c) Overflow incontinence

d) Functional incontinence

7. A pessary is:

a) A substance that is injected into tissues around the bladder opening

b) A substance that helps the bladder empty more completely

c) A common medication used to treat bladder infections

d) A stiff ring placed in the vagina

ANSWERS

1. b. False. Urinary incontinence is not a disease. It is a symptom of some other problem in the body.

2. b. False. Urinary or bladder incontinence is a common condition affecting millions of people.

3. a. True. Although urinary incontinence is more common in older people, you do not have to be elderly to be affected by it.

4. b. False. Incontinence can usually be cured, treated, or successfully managed.

5. b. False. Some types of incontinence are more common in women than in men but the condition occurs in males and females, young and old.

6. b. Electrical stimulation is used to treat both stress and urge incontinence.

7. d. A pessary is a stiff ring that is placed in the vagina.

WHEN SOMEONE IS INCONTINENT

Urinary or bladder incontinence is a common condition affecting millions of people. It involves a loss of bladder control. People with urinary incontinence are not able to hold their urine. The loss of bladder control causes a problem for the person involved and often for those close to them. You need to understand incontinence so that you can assist people affected by this condition.

Urinary incontinence may last for days, weeks or months. In some cases, it never goes away. Not being able to control urine can be very embarrassing and uncomfortable. Family and friends may even start to avoid being around the person who is incontinent.

CONSIDER FOR A MOMENT...
Have you ever cared for a person who was incontinent? If so, how do you think being incontinent affected his or her life?
How would it affect yours?

In Canada, over 1.5 million people experience incontinence. More than 13 million people in the United States and at least three million adults in the United Kingdom cannot control their bladders.

Urinary incontinence is more common in older people. Some of the changes that occur with aging may contribute to bladder problems. Urinary incontinence is not considered a "normal" part of aging, however. You do not have to be elderly to be affected by it. Incontinence occurs in males and females, young and old.

Urinary incontinence is not a disease. It is a symptom of some other problem in the body. If the person in your care appears to be incontinent, advise him to discuss his condition with a physician. Incontinence can usually be cured, treated, or successfully managed.

HOW THE NORMAL BLADDER FUNCTIONS

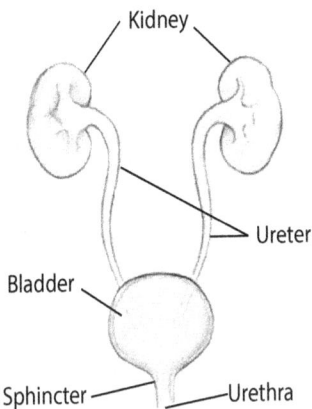

Your bladder is really a muscle. It holds the urine that your kidneys produce. The kidneys make urine all the time, day and night. Urine contains waste products and excess water from our bodies. Urine travels down tubes (called ureters) from the kidneys to the bladder a little bit at a time. We produce about two to three pints (1.5 liters) every 24 hours depending on how much we eat, drink, and sweat. As our bladders fill with urine, they expand carefully, almost like a balloon. Muscles around the bladder help prevent the urine from leaking out of the bladder outlet (urethra).

Our brains are always checking to see how full our bladders are. When the bladder starts to get full, the brain receives a message that we need to go to the bathroom. We then look for the right time and place to go to the bathroom. Most of us need to empty our bladders about four to eight times a day. Sometimes something goes "wrong" with this process. Problems develop with the brain, bladder, or muscles surrounding the bladder. Incontinence can result.

TYPES OF URINARY INCONTINENCE

Stress incontinence

The most common type of incontinence is called "stress" incontinence. This kind of stress is not the stress you feel when you are anxious or upset. The stress in stress incontinence refers to pressure that is placed on the bladder when a person coughs, sneezes, exercises, or laughs. This pressure can cause a person to leak urine if the muscles that support the bladder are weakened.

Stress incontinence is more common in women than in men. It can worsen during the week before a menstrual period because of lowered estrogen (a hormone) levels in the body. Stress incontinence is also very common during pregnancy and after childbirth. Being pregnant and the process of childbirth can put a great deal of pressure on the muscles around the bladder. The muscles can wind up quite weakened. Stress incontinence also seems to increase after menopause.

Urge incontinence

The person with urge incontinence will have a frequent, urgent need to go to the bathroom. For some people, the urge is so strong that they will not have time to get to the bathroom. Urine will leak out and they won't be able to control it. People with urge incontinence may empty their bladder in their sleep, after drinking small amounts of liquid, or even when touching water or hearing it run.

The most common cause of urge incontinence is inappropriate squeezing (contracting) of the bladder muscles (also called pelvic floor muscles). The person has no control over the contractions.

These uncontrollable contractions can occur because of damage to the bladder nerves, to the brain and spinal cord (the central nervous system), or to the bladder muscles themselves. Some diseases, such as multiple sclerosis, Parkinson's disease, Alzheimer's disease, and stroke, can harm bladder nerves or muscles. Urge incontinence can occur at any age although it is most common in men and in elderly people.

Mixed incontinence

Quite often, people find they have symptoms of both stress incontinence and urge incontinence at the same time. This is called mixed incontinence.

Functional incontinence

Functional incontinence is seen in people who have problems moving, thinking, or communicating. Older people who have trouble walking may find it impossible to get to the bathroom in time. Arthritis may make it difficult for them to undo their clothing. People with certain conditions like Alzheimer's disease may not be able to think well enough to even realize that they have to go to the bathroom. Functional incontinence is most often found in the elderly.

Overflow incontinence

You may have people in your care who constantly dribble urine. Their bladders are like a container that is constantly overflowing. They go to the bathroom but then dribble for quite some time afterwards and are not able to control it. Early symptoms of this type of incontinence include trouble with starting to pass urine. Another is an unusually slow flow of urine when they go to the bathroom.

Several conditions can cause overflow incontinence. These include weakened bladder muscles, narrowing of the urethra, tumors, constipation, and injury to the bladder or surrounding muscles. Certain conditions, such as diabetes, can cause nerve damage that weakens the bladder muscles.

Another cause of overflow incontinence is enlargement of the prostate gland in men, especially after the age of 55. The prostate gland is a fleshy organ that is wrapped around the narrow part of the bladder. If it enlarges, it can squeeze the bladder outlet until it interferes with the flow of urine out of the bladder. (Overflow incontinence is rather rare in women).

Transient incontinence

Transient incontinence is temporary. It occurs as a result of a problem or condition that will go away. The problem or condition could be an infection or a side effect of certain medications.

Nocturia

Nocturia is being woken up often at night by the need to go to the bathroom and pass urine. It is not really a type of incontinence, but can, however, be a warning of problems that are developing. Nocturia is more common over the age of 60. For instance, a normal pattern might be getting up to go to the bathroom once a night when you are in your sixties, twice a night in your seventies, three times a night in your eighties, and so on.

Nocturia has a number of possible causes. These include drinking a large amount of fluid before going to bed, the inability to hold a lot of urine as people get older, an enlarged prostate gland in older men, and excess fluid in the body.

RISK FACTORS FOR
URINARY INCONTINENCE

A number of risk factors may increase a person's chances of having urinary incontinence. These include the following:

- Some illnesses affect the way the bladder works or interfere with a person's ability to think. Examples of such conditions are stroke, diabetes, multiple sclerosis, Parkinson's disease, and Alzheimer's disease.

- Age. As a person ages, bladder muscles may weaken. In elderly men, enlargement of the prostate gland can lead to incontinence. The lack of estrogen experienced by women who have gone through menopause may make them more prone to incontinence.

- Some medications can cause incontinence or make it worse. Medications taken to rid the body of excess fluid may make a person need to go to the bathroom more often or with sudden urgency. Others taken for mental illnesses sometimes cause incontinence. Caffeine, found in coffee, tea, colas, chocolate, and some weight loss products, can make incontinence worse.

- Weakened bladder muscles and weakened muscles that surround the bladder make a person more likely to be incontinent. Obesity, injury, pregnancy, and childbirth are some of the conditions that can cause this weakness.

- Certain types of infections, such as kidney or bladder infections, increase the risk of incontinence.

- Sometimes people are incontinent because they cannot get to a bathroom fast enough. People with difficulty walking may not be able to get to the bathroom in time.

CONSIDER FOR A MOMENT...

Do you have any of the risk factors for urinary incontinence?

Do you currently care for someone with any of these risk factors?

GETTING A HISTORY

Anyone with incontinence should have a thorough examination by a doctor who is very knowledgeable about incontinence. Some types of doctors who may be able to help people with bladder problems include:

Urologist: a doctor who specializes in problems of the urinary system

Gynecologist: a doctor who specializes in women's health

Obstetrician: a doctor who specializes in childbirth

Family practice and internists: doctors who help patients with many different kinds of problems, including bladder problems

Some nurses and other healthcare workers also specialize in providing care to clients with incontinence. These professionals have special training and/or experience in working with clients who are incontinent. They are also very knowledgeable about the causes and treatment options for incontinence.

A healthcare professional will need a thorough history of a person's bladder problems. You may be asked to provide any of the following information about the person in your care as part of an overall assessment: (For our purposes, we'll assume the person is female.)

- When does the incontinence occur? During the day? At night?

- What is the person doing when she is incontinent? Coughing, laughing, exercising, or sneezing?

- How often does she pass water each day?

- How many times does she wake up at night to go to the bathroom?

- Does she feel an urgent need to rush to the bathroom?

- Does she have difficulty starting to make the urine flow?

- After going to the bathroom, does she feel as if her bladder is empty?

- Does she have to strain or push to start urine flowing?

- Does she feel pain or a burning sensation when passing water?

- Does her urine smell unpleasant?

- Is the urine an unusual color? Is there blood in it?

- How many times a day does she experience incontinence?

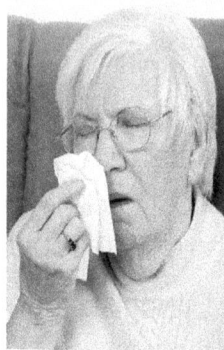

- When did the incontinence first start? How long has it been going on?
- How much urine comes out when she is incontinent? A few drops? A great deal?
- How many cups of fluid does she drink each day?
- What kinds of liquids does she drink? Do the liquids have a lot of caffeine in them?
- What medication is she taking? This includes prescription drugs, medications bought over-the-counter, vitamins, herbal supplements, and weight loss products.
- Does she have trouble walking? Is it hard to get to a bathroom? Is undressing difficult?

The answers to these and other questions, along with physical examination results, should help to identify the type of incontinence the person is experiencing and its cause.

HEALTHY BLADDER HABITS

Part of any bladder treatment program should be learning about healthy bladder habits. Below are general tips for a healthy bladder that most people can follow:

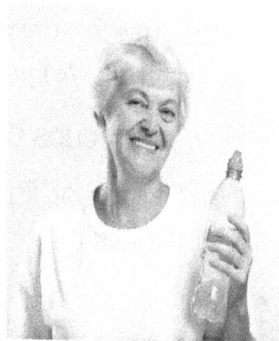

- Drink plenty of fluids, about three to four pints (two liters), per day. More fluids may be needed if the weather is hot or if you are getting lots of exercise.

- Cut back on fluids during the evening if frequent trips to the bathroom at night are a problem.

- Do not push or strain to empty the bladder.

- Cut down on alcohol and drinks that contain caffeine.

- Know when to seek medical help.

  See a doctor if you:

    o Are incontinent

    o Feel pain or burning when you go to the bathroom

    o See blood in your urine

    o Notice that your urine is an odd color

    o Notice that your urine smells foul

Encourage the people in your care to follow any specific instructions provided by their physician or other professional healthcare worker. Advise them, too, to ask questions if they do not understand the information they have been given.

TREATING URINARY INCONTINENCE

Luckily, there are many different ways of effectively treating or managing urinary incontinence. As a caregiver, you won't be responsible for deciding which method should be used but you may, however, be asked to assist with a treatment plan. These treatment methods include:

Kegel exercises

Kegel or "pelvic floor muscles" exercises are done to strengthen the muscles that help control the passing of urine. Women of all ages can learn to perform Kegel exercises to reduce or even cure stress incontinence. To locate the muscles to exercise, the person can stop and start the flow of urine when going to the bathroom. Once she understands which muscles control the passing of urine (voiding), she simply tightens and relaxes these muscles over and over.

There are many ways to perform Kegel exercises. One way is to squeeze the muscles slowly together for a few seconds and then relax them for a few seconds about 10 times several times a day. A healthcare professional should teach the person in your care how to do the exercises. She can also instruct her on how often to do them.

Vaginal cones are sometimes used with Kegel exercises. These are small weights that are placed within the vagina for short periods of time. Vaginal cones help to strengthen the muscles around the vagina.

Electrical stimulation

Brief, small doses of electrical stimulation can help to strengthen the muscles that control the flow of urine. Electrical stimulation is used to treat both stress and urge incontinence. Electrodes are placed in the vagina or rectum to stimulate the involved muscles. Most people do not feel any pain during this procedure. They may feel tingling or a tightening of the pelvic floor muscles.

Biofeedback

Biofeedback is used along with Kegel exercises and electrical stimulation to treat stress and urge incontinence in women. Biofeedback uses measuring equipment to help the person become aware of how her body functions and to gain control over bladder and pelvic muscles.

Habit training

Habit training can be helpful for people with functional incontinence. It can only be used when a normal pattern of voiding can be established. It involves taking the person to the bathroom according to the normal routine followed before the incontinence started. For example, if the person normally went to the bathroom before meals and in the middle of the morning, he or she should be taken to the bathroom at those times so that the "normal" habits are restored.

Timed voiding

To void means to urinate or pass your water. Timed voiding means that the person empties his/her bladder at specific times, often every two to four hours. This technique helps to reduce or stop incontinence and leaking. Healthcare workers caring for the elderly often follow a scheduled toileting program for certain clients who are bedridden or very frail.

Bladder retraining

Timed voiding is used with bladder retraining but the length of time between trips to the bathroom is slowly increased. In this way, the bladder trains to delay voiding for longer periods of time. This technique is sometimes used with urge and mixed incontinence.

Keeping a record

When retraining the bladder, it is helpful (and important) to keep track of information such as when the person empties his/her bladder, when incontinence occurs, and what he or she was doing when the incontinence occurred. This type of record can determine a pattern in voiding and incontinence. It can then be used to plan when to go to the bathroom to avoid being incontinent and to establish a "normal" pattern of voiding.

Medications

Medications can help to reduce incontinence. Some medications can help to relax bladder muscles. Others work in different ways to control the problem. It may take several weeks before the person notices an improvement from the medications.

Pessaries

A pessary is a stiff ring that is placed in the vagina. It presses against the wall of the vagina and the opening of the bladder. This pressure helps to lessen stress leakage. People using this device must look for possible vaginal and bladder infections and see their doctor on a regular basis.

Implants

Implants are substances that are injected into tissues around the bladder opening. These substances help to close the bladder opening and reduce stress incontinence. The injections must be repeated every so often because they do not last forever.

Surgery

Surgery is usually used only after other treatments to reduce incontinence have been tried and have failed. Many surgical procedures have high rates of success. Some common operations to assist women with stress incontinence involve lifting the neck of the bladder to help it stay closed or supporting the bladder to prevent leakage during pressure increases.

If the person in your care needs surgery, he or she should get all their questions answered before they have the surgery. A few of the issues they may want to find out about are: What exactly will be done during the operation? How long will it take to recover? When will I be able to return to work? What improvements can I expect and will these improvements last? What are the possible complications of this operation? Are they dangerous? Advise the person to write down his questions along with the answers the doctor gives him so he won't forget.

USE OF CATHETERS

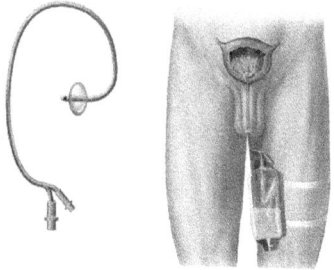

Sometimes a catheter is used to empty the bladder. This is a tube that is placed inside the bladder. It connects to a heavy plastic bag that attaches to the leg. The bag must be emptied of urine several times a day. A larger bag may be needed at night. This type of catheter is called an indwelling catheter or Foley catheter. An indwelling catheter may be left in place for days or even weeks. It needs to be changed by a healthcare professional every so often. In other words, a new tube will be placed inside the bladder and the old tube will be removed and thrown away.

If the person in your care has a chronic disorder such as a spinal cord injury, he or she may learn to do self-catheterization. In this case, the person places a catheter inside the bladder several times a day to empty it of urine. After the bladder is empty, the tube is removed right away.

Men with this condition may use a soft sleeve or condom that fits over the penis to collect urine. It may be called an external catheter, a penile sheath, or a condom catheter. It attaches to a leg drainage bag. It can be used during the day, at night, or left on for about 24 hours. Most of these devices can only be used once.

CARE CONSIDERATIONS

As we have already mentioned, incontinence is a common condition affecting millions of people. At some point in your career you will probably care for someone who is incontinent. If you work in a nursing home, chances are that a high number of your current clients are incontinent. It has been estimated that about 50% of older adults in institutions are incontinent. Incontinence is actually a common reason for admission to a nursing home.

Outlined below are a number of care considerations for you to follow as you attend to people with urinary incontinence. Some of them have been mentioned earlier in this book, but they are important enough to be mentioned again.

- Urinary incontinence can be very embarrassing and uncomfortable for the people who suffer from it, their families, and their friends. It is important to support them. Treat them with dignity and encourage them to stay active and not to avoid family and friends.

- About half the people with incontinence do not seek help for it. Encourage the people you care for to have regular physical check-ups and to report any episodes of incontinence. Teach them to keep a record of when they are incontinent and what they are doing when the incontinence takes place. Ask them to record what makes the incontinence worse and what makes it better.

- People who are incontinent may wet the bed or their clothing. They may need help to go to the bathroom because of frequent urges. Some healthcare workers may become impatient with them. They may not understand that their clients cannot control when and how often they may need to go to the bathroom. Help your co-workers understand how important it is to be supportive and not to complain or make fun of someone who is incontinent.

- Stress incontinence occurs when the person laughs, coughs, sneezes, or exercises vigorously. Women who are pregnant or have recently had children are at increased risk. They should be informed of this fact. Remember that the risk of stress incontinence increases after menopause.

- Some people have difficulty getting to the bathroom in time. It may help if their bedroom is close to a bathroom. Ensure a clear path to the bathroom. Use a night light. When someone asks for help to get to the bathroom, try to respond as soon as possible.

- People who have trouble thinking (such as those who have had a stroke or Alzheimer's disease) may not realize that they have to go to the bathroom until it is too late. Be patient with them and their loved ones. Encourage your co-workers to be patient, too.

- The people in your care should know the symptoms of bladder infections. Tell them to notify their doctor if they notice that their urine is an unusual color, has blood in it, or smells unpleasant. They should also seek medical help if they have pain or a burning sensation when they pass their urine.

- It is important to drink enough fluid every day. This will help the body get rid of waste products and prevent bladder infections. Some people who suffer from incontinence drink very little. They think that they will be incontinent less often if they drink very little. Instead, this practice increases the risk of bladder infections and other problems.

- People with incontinence should avoid alcoholic drinks and fluids (as well as other products) that contain caffeine.

- Sometimes incontinent people have trouble with starting to pass urine. Running water or stroking the inner thigh may help.

- Encourage the person to avoid drinking large amounts of fluid in the evening. This will reduce his chances of being incontinent at night or in his sleep.

- Advise the people in your care not to push or strain to empty their bladders.

- Obesity puts extra pressure on the bladder and may increase the risk of incontinence. Encourage the person to maintain her weight within a normal range for her height and age.

- Acquiring new habits is not always easy. If someone in your care is learning to perform Kegel exercises, explain that these must be done several times a day (according to the schedule developed with the doctor) for the rest of their lives.

- If people are taking prescribed medications to help treat their incontinence problems, make sure that they tell their doctors which ones they are currently taking. They should also tell their doctors about over-the-counter medications, vitamins, herbal supplements, and other supplements, such as weight loss products.

- If electrical stimulation is part of the treatment plan, explain that most people do not feel pain during this procedure. They will probably feel tingling and/or a tightening of the bladder muscles.

- Incontinent people need support and help to retrain their bladders. If someone is using a timed voiding approach, make sure that he is able to get to the bathroom when he needs to.

- If someone is using a pessary, help her to learn how to insert it, remove it, and clean it as needed.

- Surgery is a serious treatment but it is often very successful.

- Urine is very irritating to skin. If urine is left on the skin for long periods, skin breakdown can occur. Find out about the policy for skin care at your facility and follow it. If there is no specific policy, washing with mild soap and water is usually effective. Make sure the person has dry clothes to change into.

- If the person in your care has an indwelling catheter in place, wash and dry the area around the catheter carefully. Look at the urine for signs of infection and other problems such as bloody urine, cloudy urine, or urine that seems to have particles of tissue in it. You may be instructed to empty the catheter bag at regular times. When you do so, note if the urine smells unpleasant.

- Men who use an external catheter will need to wash and dry the penis carefully when changing the catheter. This will help to keep the skin free of infection and avoid skin breakdown.

- Protect beds, chairs, and other furniture from becoming soiled with urine. Bedpads can be placed on the bed under the person's waist and thighs. Covers can be used to protect mattresses, pillows, blankets, chairs, and sofas. Sometimes plastic covers are used because they can be washed and used again. These covers often become hard, however, and may split after a few washes. No matter what types of pads are used, make sure that they are removed as soon as they are soiled and clean ones put down. Wash and dry reusable pads. If the pads are to be thrown away, do so right away. Remember to help people wash and dry themselves whenever you change the pads.

- A variety of incontinence products can be worn inside a person's underwear to protect the clothing from being soiled by urine. These products are disposable. Some people prefer to use underpants that absorb urine. Some of these products are disposable. Others are washable so that they can be used more than once.

- Incontinence products vary in shape, size, and ability to absorb urine. Some work best during the day, others at night. Ensure that the person in your care uses the right product at the right time to meet his or her individual needs.

- Clothing that can be easily removed is available for people who suffer from arthritis or other similar conditions. Use of this type of clothing may allow the person to access the bathroom in time to prevent an accident from occurring.

CONSIDER FOR A MOMENT...
Can you think of other care considerations that have not already been mentioned?

CASE EXAMPLE

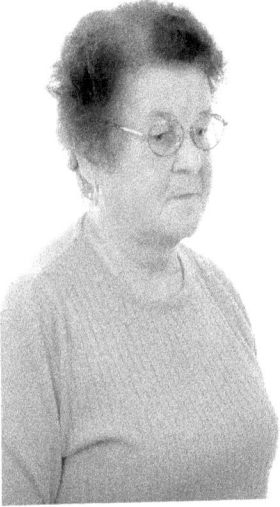

You have begun to care for Evelyn Brown who lives alone in a cluttered old house. Mrs. Brown is older woman with a number of health problems. She is easily tired and rests for most of each day. Arthritis has made her joints stiff and sore. She has to climb the stairs to reach the bathroom but she doesn't always make it in time. She sometimes has an "accident." When this happens, Mrs. Brown doesn't ask for your help.

What factors may be contributing to Mrs. Brown's "accidents"?

Is Mrs. Brown's reluctance to ask for help unusual in this situation?

What could you do to help her?

YOUR ANSWERS TO CASE EXAMPLE

SUGGESTED ANSWERS TO CASE EXAMPLE

What factors may be contributing to Mrs. Brown's "accidents"?

Based on the information given in the case example, it seems that Mrs. Brown's "accidents" may be happening because she can't get to the bathroom fast enough. Factors that may be contributing to this problem are her advanced age and fatigue, stiff joints as a result of arthritis, the presence of stairs leading to the bathroom, and clutter in the house. The clutter may be slowing her progress to the bathroom.

Is Mrs. Brown's reluctance to ask for help unusual in this situation?

No, it is not unusual. Many people with incontinence are very embarrassed by their situation.

What could you do to help her?

Some of the steps you can take to help Mrs. Brown are to:

- Gently approach the issue of incontinence. It may be helpful for Mrs. Brown to know that she is not alone. Tell her that the condition affects many people, both young and old. Reassure her. Tell her you would like to help her with her personal care needs.

- Find out if she has been assessed for her incontinence. If not, encourage her to see her physician.

- Have a discussion with Mrs. Brown about the clutter in the house. Make a plan that will ensure a clear path to the bathroom.

- Discuss the issue of the stairs. If her bedroom is downstairs, Mrs. Brown may wish to use one on an upper level to make it easier to get to the bathroom at night.

- Due to her arthritis, Mrs. Brown may find it difficult to unbutton and unzip her clothing. Find out if this is a problem for her. If so, notify your supervisor. He/she may be able to have someone knowledgeable in this area discuss clothing options with Mrs. Brown.

CONCLUSION

Incontinence is a very common problem. It affects millions of people in Canada, the United States, and the United Kingdom. It can be a frustrating and embarrassing problem not only for the person with the condition, but also for their families and their friends. People need support and encouragement as they pursue treatment.

Urinary incontinence is not a disease. It is a symptom of some type of problem within the body. Urinary incontinence can usually be cured, treated, or successfully managed. Anyone with urinary incontinence should have a thorough physical examination by a knowledgeable doctor. Treatment options include exercises, medications, and surgery. Each of these methods has advantages and disadvantages. All options should be discussed with the doctor so people can make informed choices about what treatments are best for them.

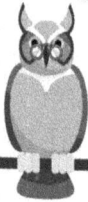

CHECK YOUR KNOWLEDGE

1. Name several types of urinary incontinence.

2. Identify the risk factors for urinary incontinence.

3. What are some general tips for a healthy bladder?

4. Identify several treatment methods for urinary incontinence.

5. Discuss care considerations for working with people who are incontinent.

TEST YOURSELF

Please circle to indicate the best answer:

1. Urinary incontinence is a normal part of aging.

a) True

b) False

2. Nearly 100% of older adults in institutions are incontinent.

a) True

b) False

3. Overflow incontinence is most common in men.

a) True

b) False

4. Kegel exercises are used to treat stress incontinence.

a) True

b) False

5. The most common type of incontinence is called:

a) Functional incontinence

b) Urge incontinence

c) Stress incontinence

d) Transient incontinence

6. Nocturia is:

a) What happens when someone has stress incontinence and urge incontinence at the same time

b) A temporary condition

c) A condition that always requires surgery to correct

d) Being woken up often at night by the need to go to the bathroom and pass urine

7. Taking someone to the bathroom according to the normal routine followed before he or she became incontinent is called:

a) Habit training

b) Timed voiding

c) Bladder retraining

d) Biofeedback

ANSWERS:

1. b. False. Urinary incontinence is not considered a "normal" part of aging – you do not have to be elderly to be affected by it.

2. b. False. It has been estimated that about 50% of older adults in institutions are incontinent.

3. a. True. In fact, overflow incontinence is rather rare in women.

4. a. True. Women of all ages can learn to perform Kegel exercises to reduce or even cure stress incontinence.

5. c. The most common type of incontinence is called "stress" incontinence.

6. d. Nocturia is being woken up often at night by the need to go to the bathroom and pass urine.

7. a. Taking someone to the bathroom according to the normal routine followed before the incontinence started is called "habit training."

REFERENCES

Bartelmo, J. M. (Ed.). (2002). Handbook of medical-surgical nursing. Springhouse, PA: Springhouse.

Edwards, P. A. (Ed.). (2000). The specialty practice of rehabilitation nursing. A core curriculum, 4th ed. Glenville, IL: Association of Rehabilitation Nursing.

Holmes, H. N. (Ed.). (2000). Handbook of diseases, 2nd ed. Springhouse, PA: Springhouse.

Houska, A. E. (Ed.). (2003). Nursing 2003 drug handbook. Philadelphia: Lippincott, Williams & Wilkins.

Hutchinson S., Leger-Krall, S. & Wilson H.S. (1996). Toileting: a biobehavioral challenge in Alzheimer's dementia care. Journal of Gerontological Nursing, 22 (10) p.18 In Potter, A. G., & Perry, P. A. (2001). Fundamentals of nursing (5th ed.). St. Louis: Mosby, Inc.

Kegel, A. H. (1948). Progressive resistance exercises in the restoration of the perineal muscles. American Journal of Obstetrics and Gynecology, pp. 238-248.

National Association for Continence. Treatment options. Retrieved December 27, 2002 http://www.nafc.org/site2/you/treatment.html.

National Kidney and Urologic Diseases Information Clearinghouse. (2002). Bladder control for women. NIH Publication No. 02-4132. Retrieved October 1, 2002 http://www.niddk.nih.gov/health/urolog/pubs/uiwomen/uiwomen.html.

Potter, A. G., & Perry, P. A. (2001). Fundamentals of nursing (5th ed.). St. Louis:Mosby, Inc.

The Canadian Continence Foundation. (2002). Facts on incontinence. Retrieved October 16, 2002 http://www.continence-fdn.ca/facts.html.

The Continence Foundation (2002). Introduction. Retrieved September 26, 2002 from http://www.continence-foundation.org.uk/symptoms-and-treatments/index.php.

The Continence Foundation (2002). Night-time problems. Retrieved September 26, 2002 http://www.continence-foundation.org.uk/symptoms-and-treatments/nighttime-problems.php.

The Continence Foundation (2002). Overflow incontinence. Retrieved September 26, 2002 from http://www.continence-foundation.org.uk/symptoms-and-treatments/overflow-incontinence.php.

The Continence Foundation (2002). Pelvic floor exercises. Retrieved September 26, 2002 from http://www.continence-foundation.org.uk/symptoms-and-treatments/pelvic-floor-exercises.php.

The Continence Foundation (2002). Stress incontinence. Retrieved September 26, 2002 from http://www.continence-foundation.org.uk/symptoms-and-treatments/stress-incontinence.php.

The Continence Foundation (2002). Surgery for success. Retrieved September 26, 2002 http://www.continence-foundation.org.uk/symptoms-and-treatments/surgery-for-stress-incontinence-in-women.php.

The Continence Foundation (2002). The healthy bladder. Retrieved September 26, 2002 http://www.continence-foundation.org.uk/symptoms-and-treatments/healthy-bladder.php.

The Continence Foundation (2002). The overactive bladder. Retrieved September 26, 2002 http://www.continence-foundation.org.uk/symptoms-and-treatments/urgency-and-frequency.php.

The Continence Foundation (2002). What can go wrong? Retrieved September 26, 2002 http://www.continence-foundation.org.uk/symptoms-and-treatments/what-can-go-wrong.php.

The Canadian Continence Foundation. (1998). Bringing incontinence out of the closet. Exploring innovative partnerships. Summary of workshop proceedings. Retrieved December 27, 2002 http://www.continence-fdn.ca/indexeng.html.